HOME WORKOUTS FOR SENIORS OVER 60

Effective Exercise Routines for Seniors' Well-Being

Johnson Myers Ella

Johnson Myers Ella

Table of Contents

Johnson Myers Ella

Home Workout for Seniors Over 60

Johnson Myers Ella

Introduction

As we age, maintaining good health becomes increasingly important, and physical exercise is one of the most effective ways to achieve this. Regular exercise can improve mobility, balance, and overall fitness, which can help to prevent falls, injuries, and chronic conditions such as heart disease, diabetes, and arthritis. For seniors over the age of 60, finding appropriate workout exercises is essential, as the body undergoes many changes with age, and not all exercises are suitable for this age group.

One inspiring story of a senior who has maintained good health with regular workouts is that of Jane. Jane is a 65-year-old woman who has been physically active her whole life. She started her fitness journey in her 20s when she joined a gym and began doing aerobics classes. Over the years, she has tried various forms of exercise, including yoga, swimming, and walking. However, when she turned 60, she noticed that her body was starting to change, and some exercises were becoming more difficult.

After consulting with her doctor, Jane learned that her bone density was decreasing, and she was at risk of osteoporosis. Her doctor recommended that she incorporate weight-bearing exercises into her routine to strengthen her bones. Jane decided to join a strength training class at her local gym, where she learned how to use weights and resistance bands to build muscle and increase bone density.

At first, Jane found the exercises challenging, and she was sore for several days after each class. However, with persistence and determination, she began to see improvements

Johnson Myers Ella

in her strength and balance. She was also pleased to discover that her bone density had increased, reducing her risk of osteoporosis.

Now, five years later, Jane is still attending her strength training class twice a week. She has also started doing gentle yoga and walking regularly to maintain her flexibility and cardiovascular health. She is proud of the progress she has made and is grateful for the many benefits of regular exercise, including increased energy, better sleep, and improved mood.

Jane's story is a testament to the importance of regular exercise for seniors over 60. It highlights the need for appropriate workout exercises that take into account the changes that occur in the body with age. As we age, our muscles weaken, our bones become more fragile, and our joints may become stiff and

Johnson Myers Ella

painful. Therefore, it is essential to choose exercises that are safe, effective, and enjoyable.

Many workout exercises for seniors over 60 can help to improve mobility, balance, strength, and flexibility. Some of these exercises include low-impact aerobics, yoga, Tai Chi, strength training, and water aerobics. Each of these exercises has its benefits and can be adapted to suit individual needs and abilities.

In conclusion, regular exercise is essential for maintaining good health and preventing chronic conditions in seniors over 60. Jane's story is an inspiring example of the benefits of regular exercise, and it highlights the importance of choosing appropriate workout exercises for this age group. With the right exercise routine, seniors can improve their physical and mental health, increase their energy and vitality, and enjoy a better quality of life.

Johnson Myers Ella

Chapter One

Introducing Workouts

Workouts are physical exercises or activities that are performed to improve or maintain physical fitness and overall health. Workouts can take many forms, including cardiovascular exercises such as running or cycling, strength training exercises such as weight lifting, and flexibility exercises such as yoga or stretching. Workouts can be tailored to meet individual fitness goals and can be performed individually or in a group setting. The intensity and duration of workouts can vary depending on individual fitness levels, health status, and personal preferences. Workouts are an important component of a healthy lifestyle and can help to prevent chronic conditions such as heart disease, diabetes, and obesity, among others.

Importance of Exercise for Seniors

Exercise is essential for people of all ages, but it becomes increasingly important as we age. For seniors, regular exercise is critical for maintaining physical and mental health, preventing chronic conditions, and improving quality of life. Here are some of the reasons why exercise is so important for seniors:

Maintaining Strength and Balance

As we age, we naturally lose muscle mass and bone density, which can lead to weakness and increased risk of falls. Regular exercise, especially strength training and balance exercises, can help to maintain muscle mass and bone density, improving strength and balance.

Johnson Myers Ella

Improving Cardiovascular Health

Exercise, especially aerobic exercise, can help to improve cardiovascular health by reducing blood pressure, improving circulation, and lowering cholesterol levels.

Managing Chronic Conditions

Exercise can help to manage and prevent a variety of chronic conditions that are common among seniors, including diabetes, arthritis, and heart disease. Exercise can help to reduce inflammation, improve glucose control, and improve overall health and well-being.

Improving Mental Health

Exercise is an effective way to reduce symptoms of depression and anxiety, which are common among seniors. Cognitive function can be improved through exercise.

Johnson Myers Ella

Increasing Independence

By improving strength, balance, and mobility, regular exercise can help seniors maintain their independence and reduce the risk of needing assistance with activities of daily living.

Social Benefits

Exercise can be a social activity, providing opportunities for seniors to connect with others and reduce social isolation, which is a risk factor for many health problems.

Improving Sleep

Exercise can improve sleep quality and reduce the risk of insomnia, which is common among seniors.

Overall, regular exercise is crucial for maintaining physical and mental health, preventing chronic conditions, and improving the quality of life for seniors. Seniors should

Johnson Myers Ella

consult with their healthcare provider before starting any exercise program and should choose exercises that are appropriate for their fitness level and health status.

Exercise Guidelines for Seniors with Health Issues

Seniors must regularly exercise to preserve their physical and mental health, but several health issues must be taken into mind. The following are some important health factors for seniors exercising:

Medical History

Before beginning an exercise program, seniors should speak with their healthcare practitioner about their medical history, as well as any ailments or injuries that could limit their ability to exercise safely.

Cardiovascular Health

Seniors should exercise with care if they have a history of heart disease, high blood pressure, or other cardiovascular disorders. While exercising, it's crucial to keep an eye on your heart rate and blood pressure and steer clear of anything that can be overly demanding.

Joint Health

To prevent aggravating joint discomfort, seniors with arthritis or other joint disorders may need to change their activity regimen. For seniors with joint issues, low-impact workouts like walking, swimming, and cycling might be beneficial.

Seniors who are in danger of falling or who have mobility problems should concentrate on activities that boost balance and mobility, including tai chi or yoga. To lower the chance of falls, it's necessary to take measures like

Johnson Myers Ella

using a cane or walker or working out with a partner.

14

Medication

Some medicines may make it more difficult for an elderly person to exercise safely. Seniors should speak with their doctor to find out if any drugs they are taking might make it more difficult for them to exercise properly.

Seniors are more prone to heat-related illnesses, therefore it is crucial to exercise in a cool atmosphere and to drink enough water.

Fatigue

Older folks may tire more quickly than younger ones, so it's crucial to begin an exercise program at a lesser intensity and gradually increase it as your fitness level rises.

Johnson Myers Ella

Recovery

Seniors may need longer recovery periods in between exercises, so it's vital to pay attention to your body and take it easy when you need to.

In general, elders should exercise prudence and be aware of any health issues or physical restrictions. Seniors should speak with their healthcare professionals before beginning any new exercise program since fitness levels and health conditions should be taken into account when designing an exercise program. Seniors may exercise safely and successfully to enhance their physical and mental health by taking these health issues into mind.

Pre-existing Conditions to Take Into Account

Before beginning an exercise program, seniors should be evaluated for any underlying medical

Johnson Myers Ella

issues that could limit their capacity to exercise safely. Here are some typical medical problems to take into account:

Cardiovascular Disease

Seniors should exercise with extra care if they have a history of heart disease, high blood pressure, or other cardiovascular disorders. While exercising, it's crucial to keep an eye on your heart rate and blood pressure and steer clear of anything that can be overly demanding.

Arthritis

To prevent aggravating joint discomfort, seniors who have arthritis or other joint disorders may need to change their exercise regimen. For seniors with joint issues, low-impact workouts like walking, swimming, and cycling might be beneficial.

Johnson Myers Ella

Osteoporosis

Seniors with poor bone density or osteoporosis may need to change their exercise regimen to stay away from activities that raise their risk of fracture. Strength training or weight-bearing activities like walking may help to enhance bone density, but it's crucial to utilize appropriate techniques and stay away from high-impact exercises that might raise your chance of being hurt.

Diabetes

Seniors who have the disease may need to regularly check their blood sugar levels while exercising and modify their insulin or prescription dosages as necessary. Exercise may aid in better glucose regulation, but it's crucial to avoid working out when blood sugar levels are abnormally low or high.

Johnson Myers Ella

Seniors with chronic obstructive pulmonary disease (COPD) may need to alter their exercise regimen to prevent aggravating breathing problems. Seniors with COPD might benefit from exercises that increase cardiovascular fitness, such as walking or cycling, but it's vital to start with low-intensity workouts and steer clear of activities that make you gasp for air.

Cancer

Depending on the kind and stage of their cancer, seniors with a history of the disease may need to change their exercise regimen. During and after cancer treatment, exercise may help to increase strength and decrease tiredness, but it's vital to speak with a healthcare professional before beginning an exercise program.

Seniors should, in general, speak with their healthcare professionals before beginning an exercise program to go through any pre-existing

Johnson Myers Ella

medical concerns or limits that may impair their ability to exercise safely. Seniors may create an exercise regimen that is safe and suitable for their particular requirements by considering these factors.

Screening Before Workout

Seniors should get a pre-exercise assessment before beginning a program to determine their physical fitness for exercise and spot any possible health dangers. Before beginning an exercise, elders should have the following pre-existing tests completed:

Physical Examination

To determine their general health state and spot any underlying medical disorders that can limit their ability to exercise safely, seniors should get a comprehensive physical checkup.

Johnson Myers Ella

Medical History

A study of the senior's medical history might reveal any recurring illnesses that may call for extra care when exercising, such as diabetes, high blood pressure, or heart disease.

Cardiovascular Risk Assessment

A cardiovascular risk assessment may assist identify elderly citizens who may have a higher risk of developing heart disease or stroke, and it can also help establish if any special exercise safety measures are required.

Functional Fitness Evaluation

A functional fitness evaluation may spot any physical restrictions or functional deficits that can make it more difficult for the elderly person to exercise sensibly and successfully.

A balance and mobility exam may assist identify elders who are at risk of falling or who have mobility issues, and it can also help establish if any particular exercises or safety measures should be implemented to lower the risk of falls.

Bone Density Evaluation

A bone density evaluation helps identify elderly people who are at risk for osteoporosis or bone fractures and help establish if any safety measures should be taken while exercising.

Psychological Evaluation

A psychological evaluation helps identify seniors who may be vulnerable to depression or anxiety and assist establish if exercise can be utilized as a form of treatment.

Pre-exercise screening may generally assist in identifying any possible health concerns or restrictions that may influence a senior's capacity for safe and efficient activity. Seniors

Johnson Myers Ella

may create an exercise regimen that is safe and suited to their specific requirements by undertaking pre-exercise screening.

Changes to Accommodate Particular Demands

Exercise program adaptations for special needs are developed to suit people with physical or mental impairments, accidents, ongoing medical problems, or other unique requirements. Making physical activity safe, usable, and accessible for persons with a range of needs and abilities is the aim of exercise modifications. Here are a few instances of adaptations to exercises for people with specific needs:

Adaptations to the Exercise environment

To accommodate people with physical impairments, the exercise environment may need to be changed. This may include adding wheelchair ramps, changing the equipment, or offering transfer support.

Exercise equipment modifications may be necessary to accommodate people with physical impairments, such as switching from weights to resistance bands or utilizing special grips for those with hand or wrist difficulties.

Exercise intensity adjustments may be necessary to accommodate people with chronic medical issues. For example, the length or intensity of the exercise program may need to be decreased, or rest periods may need to be added as necessary.

Modification of Exercise Type

Low-impact activities or modifications to exercises to lower the risk of harm may be necessary to accommodate those with physical or cognitive limitations.

Johnson Myers Ella

Include Assistive Equipment

To aid those with mobility or balance issues, an exercise program may include assistive equipment such as canes, walkers, or braces.

Using Visual or Verbal Clues

People with cognitive or sensory impairments may benefit from using visual or verbal cues to assist them to grasp the activity and follow directions.

Include Social Support

Social support, such as working out with a spouse or in a group, may aid people with disabilities or long-term medical issues in maintaining their motivation and interest in exercise.

The goal of exercise adaptations for special needs is to make physical activity accessible, secure, and efficient for people with a wide

Johnson Myers Ella

range of requirements and abilities. Individuals may benefit from exercise's physical, emotional, and social advantages regardless of their capabilities or limitations by making accommodations for particular requirements.

The Significance of Diet and Hydration

Any fitness plan must include both nutrition and hydration, particularly for elderly citizens. The following are some major reasons why seniors should stay hydrated and eat well when exercising:

Seniors are more susceptible to dehydration owing to age-related changes in the body's capacity to control fluid balance. Proper hydration helps maintain body temperature. A senior's risk of overheating during activity might be increased by dehydration, which helps control body temperature.

Seniors need enough energy to power their exercises, and nutrient-dense diets provide the essential carbs, proteins, and fats to promote energy metabolism during exercise.

Seniors require enough protein to maintain their muscles' health and avoid muscle loss, which may happen as people become older. Consuming enough protein before and after exercise may boost muscle development and repair.

Proper hydration and nutrition improve cognitive function. This is crucial for seniors who may be at risk of cognitive decline since it may support cognitive performance during activity.

Johnson Myers Ella

Electrolytes Help Maintain Fluid Balance

Sodium and potassium, two electrolytes, are crucial for maintaining fluid balance and healthy muscular function. Getting enough electrolytes while exercising may help avoid cramping and dehydration.

Proper Diet and Hydration Promote Immune Function

Seniors, who may have compromised immune systems, should pay special attention to proper nutrition and hydration as these two factors may support immune function.

Healing is Aided by Proper Hydration and Nutrition After Exercise

This is crucial for seniors, who may take longer to recover from exercise since it helps lessen muscular pain and promote healing.

Johnson Myers Ella

Nutrition and hydration are essential parts of any exercise plan, particularly for seniors. Seniors may be more active and healthy by maintaining proper hydration and nutrition, which can improve energy metabolism, muscular health, cognitive function, immunological function, and recuperation.

Johnson Myers Ella

Johnson Myers Ella

Chapter Two

Senior Exercise Options

Elderly people over the age of 60 may benefit from a variety of workouts. Strength, flexibility, balance, and general physical health may all be enhanced by these activities, which can also have a favorable impact on mental health and wellness. The following exercise categories are especially advantageous for seniors:

Strength Training

To increase and maintain muscle mass and strength, strength training exercises are performed using weights, resistance bands, or just one's body weight. Seniors may preserve functional independence and lower their risk of falls and fractures by engaging in strength training.

Exercises that raise heart rate and respiration, such as brisk walking, cycling, or swimming, are considered cardiovascular exercises. Cardiovascular exercise may increase general fitness and endurance while lowering the risk of chronic illnesses and improving heart health.

Exercises for Balance

Balance exercises comprise movements that test stability and balance, including standing on one leg or walking heel-to-toe. Exercises that increase balance and coordination may lower the chance of falling.

Exercises for Flexibility

Stretching and lengthening muscles and joints during flexibility exercises may increase the range of motion and lower the chance of injury. Popular senior flexibility exercises include Pilates and yoga.

Johnson Myers Ella

Exercises that may be done while sitting in a chair are known as "chair exercises." Because they are low-impact exercises, seniors with mobility or balance concerns can execute them. Balance, flexibility, and strength may all be improved with chair exercises.

Workouts in The Water

Because of the buoyancy of the water, workouts in the water, such as swimming or water aerobics, might be advantageous for seniors. Strength, flexibility, and cardiovascular health may all be enhanced with water activities.

Seniors over the age of 60 may benefit from a wide variety of workouts. Before beginning a new exercise program, it is crucial to pick activities that are suitable for your fitness level and health problems. You should also speak with your healthcare professional. Seniors may maintain their independence, health, and activity by including a variety of activities in a regular fitness schedule.

Cardiological Training

Workouts that raise heart rate and breathing are known as cardiovascular workouts, and they are especially helpful for enhancing heart health, lowering the risk of chronic illnesses, and enhancing general fitness and endurance. Here is a thorough rundown of a few well-liked cardiovascular activities for those over 60:

Walking

The majority of seniors may easily obtain this low-impact type of cardiovascular exercise. Walking may be adapted to match different fitness levels and can be done outside, on a treadmill, or in a walking group. Walking briskly for at least 30 minutes each day may help decrease blood pressure, enhance cardiovascular health, and minimize the chance

Johnson Myers Ella

of developing chronic illnesses including diabetes, heart disease, and stroke.

Swimming

Seniors who have joint discomfort or arthritis might benefit greatly from this low-impact cardiovascular activity. Water's buoyancy lessens the strain on joints and muscles while providing resistance to increase strength and stamina. Swimming may lower the chance of developing chronic illnesses, strengthen muscles, and enhance cardiovascular health.

Cycling

This is a low-impact aerobic workout that may be performed either outside or on a stationary cycle. Cycling may lower the chance of developing chronic illnesses, strengthen the legs, and enhance cardiovascular health. Cycling may be tailored to specific fitness

Johnson Myers Ella

levels by changing the resistance or length, for example.

Dancing

Dancing may be tailored to accommodate individual fitness levels and tastes. It's a fun and sociable type of cardiovascular training. Cardiovascular, balance, coordination, and mental health may all be enhanced by dancing. For older adults, popular dance-based cardiovascular activities include line dancing, ballroom dancing, and Zumba.

Running, jumping, or high-intensity interval training (HIIT) are examples of workouts that employ a lot of major muscle groups and continuous activity. Aerobic exercise may lower the chance of developing chronic illnesses, strengthen the body and increase endurance. Step aerobics and water aerobics are examples

Johnson Myers Ella

of low-impact aerobics that may be tailored to each person's degree of fitness.

Cardiovascular workouts may assist seniors to increase their general health and well-being, lowering their chance of developing chronic illnesses and enhancing their overall fitness. Before beginning a new exercise program, it is crucial to pick activities that are suitable for your fitness level and health problems. You should also speak with your healthcare professional.

Exercises for Building Strength

Squats

Squats are a fantastic strength-training exercise that may help seniors gain more stability, balance, and strength in their lower body. Here is a detailed tutorial on how to do squats safely and successfully for seniors:

Johnson Myers Ella

To begin, place your feet hip-width apart and point your toes forward. For balance, stretch your hands in front of you or place them on your hips.

After taking a breath, bend your knees and push your hips back to start lowering your body. Raise your chest and maintain a straight back

As far as is comfortable for you, lower your body till your thighs are parallel to the floor. Ensure that your knees do not protrude beyond your toes.

Take a deep breath out, and raise your body back up to a standing posture by pushing through your heels. As you rise, be sure to contract your glutes and your core.

Johnson Myers Ella

You should execute the exercise 8–12 times, or as many as you can easily do while maintaining proper form.

Advice on good form:

- Keep your feet level on the floor the whole time you are exercising.
- Do not allow your knees to fold inward; instead, keep them parallel to your toes.
- Raise your chest and maintain a straight back
- Keep your core muscles active, all through the workout.
- Don't hold your breath, and breathe in and out after each repeat.

Modifications:

- If necessary, hold on to a chair or other sturdy object for balance.
- Squat depth should be adjusted to a comfortable level.

Johnson Myers Ella

- To make the workout harder, use weights or a resistance band.

Taking Safety Into Account

Before engaging in any lower body activity, seniors with knee or hip issues should speak with a healthcare professional.

- To avoid injury, always warm up before beginning any workout regimen and stretch afterward.

- Stop the workout right once and see a doctor if you feel any pain or discomfort while doing it.

Squats may help seniors preserve their independence, improve balance, and lower their risk of fractures and falls by including them in a regular strength training program. It's crucial, to begin with a manageable number of repetitions and progressively increase the exercise's intensity and length over time.

Johnson Myers Ella

Lunges

Lunges are a fantastic strength-training activity that may help seniors gain more stability, balance, and strength in their lower bodies. A step-by-step instruction manual for doing lunges safely and successfully is provided below:

To begin, place your feet hip-width apart and point your toes forward. For balance, stretch your hands in front of you or place them on your hips.

Keep your left foot where it is and advance with your right foot. By bending your right knee and pulling your hips back, you may lower your body. Raise your chest while your back remains straight.

As far as it is comfortable for you, lower your body till your right thigh is parallel to the floor.

Check to see that your right knee does not touch your toes.

To raise your body back to a standing posture, exert pressure via your right heel. As you rise, be sure to contract your glutes and your core.

Take a big stride forward and bend your left knee to lower your torso while you repeat the motion with your left foot.

Repeat the exercise with alternate legs for 8–12 repetitions, or as many as you can comfortably complete while maintaining proper form.

Tips for proper conduct:

- Keep your feet flat on the floor during the whole workout.
- Don't allow your knees to bend inward; keep them parallel to your toes.

Johnson Myers Ella

- Raise your chest, and maintain a straight back

- Utilize your core muscles consistently throughout the workout.

- Take a regular, in-and-out breath after each repetition.

Modifications:

- If necessary, cling to a chair or other sturdy object for balance.

- Pick a step length that seems natural to you.

- To make the workout harder, use weights or a resistance band.

Considering Safety

- Before doing lunges or any other lower body exercise, seniors with knee or hip issues should see a doctor.

- To avoid injury, always warm up before beginning any workout program and stretch afterward.
- Stop exercising right once and see a doctor if you experience any pain or discomfort.

Seniors may be able to preserve their independence, improve their balance, and lower their risk of fractures and falls by including lunges in a regular strength training regimen. It's crucial, to begin with a manageable number of repetitions and progressively build up the exercise's length and intensity over time.

Wall Pushups

Push-ups against a wall are fantastic exercises for seniors to increase upper-body stability and strength. The elderly may safely and properly do wall pushups by watching the video that follows:

Johnson Myers Ella

Find a solid wall so you can press your hands against it. Stand with your feet shoulder-width apart and approximately an arm's length away from the wall.

Lay flat against the wall with your hands shoulder-width apart. Your fingers ought to be pointing up.

Constrict your core muscles while you lean forward just a little bit. Stand straight.

Lower your chest toward the wall while bending your elbows. Hold your neck in a neutral posture and keep your back straight.

To straighten your arms and go back to the beginning position, push through your hands. As you push back, be careful to contract your triceps and compress your chest.

Johnson Myers Ella

The exercise should be completed 8–12 times or as many as you can manage with the appropriate form.

Advice on appropriate behavior
- Throughout the whole workout, keep your elbows tight to your torso.
- Hold your neck in a neutral posture and keep your back straight.
- To keep your body in the proper position, contract your abdominal muscles.
- Take a regular, in-and-out breath after each repetition.

Modifications:
- Change the distance between you and the wall to adjust the exercise's difficulty.
- If required, place your hands away from the wall on a stable surface, such as a table or countertop.

Johnson Myers Ella

- To make the workout harder, use weights or a resistance band.

Considering safety

- Before engaging in any upper body activity, seniors with back or shoulder issues should consult with a healthcare professional.
- To avoid injury, always warm up before beginning any workout program and stretch afterward.
- Stop exercising right once and see a doctor if you experience any pain or discomfort.

A senior's strength training program may benefit from the inclusion of wall push-ups to help them preserve their independence and develop upper body strength. It's crucial, to begin with a manageable number of repetitions

Johnson Myers Ella

and progressively build up the exercise's length and intensity over time.

Using A Bench Press

Seniors may increase their arm strength and bicep tone by doing bicep curls, a common strength training activity. The steps listed below will show you how to do bicep curls safely and effectively:

With your feet shoulder-width apart and your knees slightly bent, stand or sit comfortably.

With your arms at your sides, hold a set of dumbbells or other weighted items in your hands, palms up.

Contract your abdominal muscles, and keep your back straight and

Bend your elbows while maintaining your wrists straight and gradually bringing the weights up to your shoulders.

When the workout reaches its peak, pause briefly and squeeze your biceps.

Straighten your elbows and wrists as you gradually restore the weights to their starting position.

The exercise should be completed 8–12 times or as many as you can manage with the appropriate form.

Advice on appropriate behavior:

- Throughout the whole workout, keep your elbows tight to your torso.
- As you raise the weights, keep your wrists straight and avoid twisting them.

Johnson Myers Ella

- To keep your body in the proper position, contract your abdominal muscles.
- It is not acceptable to elevate or swing the weights.

Modifications:

- To alter the level of difficulty of the activity, use lower weights or resistance bands.
- If you have trouble raising both weights at once, try lifting one arm at a time.
- Sit down on a bench or chair if standing is unpleasant or difficult.

Safety

Seniors with shoulder or elbow problems should see a healthcare provider before doing bicep curls or any other upper-body exercise.

- Always warm up before starting any exercise program, and stretch afterward, to prevent injury.

Johnson Myers Ella

- If you have any pain or discomfort while exercising, stop immediately and visit a doctor.

By including bicep curls in a regular strength training routine, elderly persons may be able to maintain their independence and strengthen their arms. It's important to start with a weight that feels comfortable and raise the weight and repetitions gradually as you go.

Leg Curls

Seniors may benefit from strengthening their legs with leg curls, which are a terrific workout for hamstring development. A step-by-step instruction manual for doing leg curls safely and successfully is provided below:

With your legs straight and toes pointing down, lie face down on a bench or workout mat.

While maintaining your thigh on the mat or seat, bend one leg at the knee and gently bring your foot toward your buttocks.

At the peak of the exercise, pause briefly and tighten your hamstring.

Take your foot back slowly to the starting position.

After 8 to 12 repetitions, swap legs and continue the workout.

Advice on good form:

- Throughout the exercise, maintain a constant hip and upper body position.
- As you elevate your foot, concentrate on tightening your hamstring.
- To activate your hamstring muscles, maintain a downward toe-pointing position.

Johnson Myers Ella

- As you elevate your foot, try not to arch your lower back.

Modifications:

- To change the level of difficulty of the workout, use ankle weights or resistance bands.
- If you need more support, hold onto a solid object like a bench or chair.
- If reclining facedown while the exercise makes you uncomfortable, do it while sitting.

Safety

- Before exercising leg curls or any other lower body exercise, seniors with knee or back issues should speak with a healthcare professional.
- To avoid injury, always warm up before beginning any workout regimen and stretch afterward.

Johnson Myers Ella

- Stop the workout right once and see a doctor if you feel any pain or discomfort while doing it.

Seniors may increase their balance, mobility, and general leg strength by doing leg curls in a regular strength training program. Starting with a comfortable range of motion is crucial, and the number of repetitions and sets should be increased gradually over time.

Weightlifting

Seniors may benefit greatly from the popular strength-training practice known as weight lifting. Here is a step-by-step instruction for seniors on safe and efficient weight lifting:

Pick a weight that you can lift and hold comfortably. Starting at 2 to 5 pounds is an excellent idea.

Johnson Myers Ella

With your knees slightly bent and your core engaged, stand with your feet shoulder-width apart.

With your palms facing inward and your arms outstretched at your sides, hold the weight firmly in both hands.

Bend your elbows and raise the weight slowly toward your chest while maintaining your arms close to your torso.

At the peak of the exercise, pause briefly and clench your biceps.

Return the weight to its initial position by lowering it gradually.

The exercise should be repeated 8–12 times.

Johnson Myers Ella

Advice on good form:

- Throughout the workout, keep your shoulders down and your back straight.
- To raise the weight, pay attention to utilizing your biceps rather than your shoulders or back.
- Exhale as you raise the weight, and inhale as you decrease it.
- Move slowly throughout the whole workout

Modifications:

- If bigger weights are too difficult, try using lower weights or resistance bands.
- If standing while the workout is bothersome, do it while sitting.
- If necessary, use a weight bench as support.

Johnson Myers Ella

Safety

Before doing weight lifting or any other strength training activity, seniors with joint issues or other health issues should speak with a healthcare professional.

- To avoid injury, always warm up before beginning any workout regimen and stretch afterward.
- Stop the workout right once and see a doctor if you feel any pain or discomfort while doing it.

Seniors may increase their upper body strength, posture, and total muscle mass by adding weight lifting to a regular strength training program. It's crucial to start with a weight that feels comfortable and gradually raise the weight as your power grows.

Johnson Myers Ella

Yoga

Yoga is a kind of physical activity that may enhance balance, flexibility, and strength. Here is a step-by-step instruction on how elders may use yoga as a type of strength training safely and effectively:

Pick a yoga practice that strengthens a particular muscle area, such as the Warrior II stance for stronger legs or the Plank pose for stronger core muscles.

Warm up first to get your body ready for the exercise. Muscles and joints may be made more flexible with the aid of gentle stretches like shoulder shrugs and neck rolls.

Observe the proper alignment for the yoga posture you have selected. For instance:

Standing with your feet hip-width apart and your arms outstretched is the Warrior II position.

Slightly turn your right foot in and let your left foot out.

Bend your left knee and cross your left leg with your arms. After several breaths in the position, turn sides.

Start in the push-up position with your feet hip-width apart and your hands shoulder-width apart. Hold your body in a straight line from head to heels by contracting your core muscles. For many breaths, maintain the position.

Hold the posture for several breaths or do the yoga pose 8–12 times.

Johnson Myers Ella

Advice on good form:

- Pay attention to your breathing as you deepen the stretch and keep your balance.
- To maintain stability, keep your body straight and contract your core muscles.
- Throughout the position, move with control and slowness.

Modifications:

- To maintain stability or balance, use a chair or another support.
- If a position is too difficult, support yourself with a block or bolster.
- If the position is too difficult, shorten its time or the number of repetitions.

Taking safety into account

- Before engaging in yoga or any other kind of exercise, seniors with joint issues or other health issues should speak with a healthcare professional.

- To avoid injury, always warm up before beginning any workout regimen and stretch afterward.
- When doing the position, stop immediately and seek medical advice if you feel any pain or discomfort.

Seniors may increase their general muscle mass, balance, and coordination by including yoga in a regular strength training program. Starting with poses that are suitable for your level of fitness is crucial, and as your strength develops over time, you should progressively increase the intensity of the postures.

Pilates

Pilates is a kind of exercise that emphasizes using regulated movements to increase body awareness, flexibility, and strength. Here is a step-by-step explanation of how seniors may use Pilates as a kind of strength training safely and efficiently:

Pick a Pilates exercise that strengthens a particular muscle area, such as the Pilates push-up for the upper body or the side leg lift for the lower body.

Warm up first to get your body ready for the exercise. You may relax your muscles and joints while focusing on your body with the aid of gentle stretches and breathing exercises.

Be sure you do the Pilates exercise you have selected with the proper form. For instance:

Start in a plank posture with your feet hip-width apart and your hands shoulder-width apart.

Lower your body toward the floor while keeping your elbows close to your sides. Start from the beginning position by pushing up. Continue to repeat multiple times.

Lie on your side with your feet flexed and your legs straight. Your upper leg should be raised to hip height and then lowered again.

Hold the stance for several breaths or do the Pilates exercise 8–12 times.

Advice on good form:
- Pay attention to your breathing as you deepen the stretch and keep your balance.
- To maintain stability, keep your body straight and contract your core muscles.
- Throughout the whole workout, move softly and under control.

Johnson Myers Ella

Modifications:

- If you need balance or stability, use a resistance band or another kind of support.
- If a position is too difficult, support yourself with a yoga block or cushion.
- If the exercise is too difficult, shorten its time or repetition count.

Safety

- Before engaging in Pilates or any other exercise, seniors with joint issues or other health issues should speak with a healthcare professional.
- To avoid injury, always warm up before beginning any workout regimen and stretch afterward.
- Stop the workout right once and see a doctor if you feel any pain or discomfort while doing it.

Johnson Myers Ella

Seniors may increase their general muscle mass, balance, and coordination by including Pilates in a regular strength training program. It is crucial, to begin with activities that are suitable for your current level of fitness and to progressively raise the complexity of the workouts as your strength increases over time.

Exercises for Flexibility and Balance

Flexibility and balance are essential elements of senior fitness. The following balance and flexibility exercises are suitable for seniors:

Tai Chi

This is a Chinese martial art and is often practiced for its healing effects. It requires steady, flowing actions and is completed standing up. Tai chi is a fantastic kind of exercise for seniors since it improves their balance, flexibility, and strength.

Here is a detailed illustration of how a senior may do Tai Chi:

Start your warm-up by standing with your feet shoulder-width apart and your arms at your sides. Relax your body and take a breath. Gently raise your arms to shoulder height, then gently lower them again. Repeat this many times.

Raise your left foot and advance with a forward stride starting from the starting position. Your weight should now be on your left foot while you raise your right heel off the ground. With your palms facing down, Place your arms out in front of you. Holding this position for a moment, step back with your right foot to return to your starting position. Turn to the other side, and repeat this movement.

Johnson Myers Ella

Moving forward with your left foot while transferring your weight from your right foot to your left foot is the second motion. After elevating your right knee to the side, lower it back down. Your right foot should be lowered as you lift the left heel off the floor. Spread your arms out to the sides with your hands down. After a little period of holding this stance, take a left footstep back and then return to your starting position. Turn to the other side, and repeat this movement.

Stepping forward with your left foot while transferring your weight from your right foot to your left foot is the third movement. Lift your right foot and out to the side, step down with it, and shift your weight to it. As you pivot with your left foot and shift your weight to your right foot, lift your left heel off the ground. Palms should be facing down and arms should be at the sides. Right-turn your whole body. After a little period of holding this stance, take a left footstep back and then return to your starting position. Turn to the other side, and repeat this movement.

To finish your Tai Chi session, unwind by letting your body relax and taking a few deep breaths. Exercise your legs and arms to release any tension.

Tips and Modifications:
- Start with simple exercises and gradually increase their difficulty as your flexibility and balance improve.
- Use a chair or similar balance device if required.
- Practice Tai Chi in a calm, quiet environment to help you focus on your movements.

Johnson Myers Ella

- If you have any health concerns, see your doctor before starting Tai Chi.
- You may practice tai chi by yourself or with others.

Standing on a Foot

Standing on one foot is a simple yet effective balance exercise for seniors. It may be carried out anytime and whenever without the need for particular equipment. Here is a detailed illustration of how a senior may do this exercise:

Find a sturdy item, like a chair or a wall, to hold onto for support. Stand upright with your feet hip-width apart.

Lift one foot off the ground while keeping your knee slightly bent.

If it takes you that long to keep balanced, hold this position for 10 to 30 seconds.

Bring your foot to the ground and for the other side, repeat the same.

Advice and Alterations:

- Start by holding onto a stable object until you feel more comfortable and secure in your ability to balance.
- If you have trouble lifting one foot off the ground, consider shifting your weight to that foot while lifting the other foot just a little bit.
- To make the exercise more challenging, try closing your eyes while standing on one foot or holding a little amount of weight in one hand.
- It's important to breathe normally during this exercise without holding your breath.
- Make sure you switch between the two feet to maintain your equilibrium and strength on both sides of your body.

Johnson Myers Ella

Heel to Toe Stride

A balance exercise that may help with coordination and flexibility is walking from heel to toe. Here is a detailed illustration of how a senior may do this exercise:

Look for a level area where you have room to take a few steps, such as a hallway or an open area. Put your feet together firmly and stand tall.

Step forward with your right foot while keeping your left foot on the ground until your right heel is directly in front of your left foot's toes and almost touching.

As you go forward with your left foot, your left heel should be directly in front of your right foot's toes.

Place the heel of one foot directly in front of the toes of the other foot and continue doing this for 10–20 steps.

You are allowed to utilize a sturdy item for support, such as a chair or a wall, if necessary.

Advice and Alterations:

- Take small steps at first, then go gently until you feel confident in your ability to keep your balance.

- Since it is a walk, look straight ahead rather than down at your feet since this may help with balance and coordination.

- When walking, be mindful to maintain a steady pace and a straight line with your feet.

- If you're having problems, try widening the distance between your feet or holding onto a solid object while you do this exercise.

Johnson Myers Ella

- To make the exercise more difficult, consider walking backward or on a narrow surface, such as a balance board or a line on the ground.

Leg Swings

Leg swings are a quick and efficient exercise that may help seniors gain flexibility and balance. Here is a thorough example of how to carry out this exercise:

Find a stable object to grab onto for support, such as a chair or a wall. With your feet shoulder-width apart and your hands supporting you, stand up straight.

Then, swing your right leg back as far as you can while keeping your left foot firmly planted on the ground. Imagine that you are attempting to touch your toes to the wall in front of you.

After doing this motion 10 to 15 times with one leg, repeat with the other leg.

Advice and Changes

- As your balance and flexibility improve, progressively increase the height and range of your leg swings by beginning with a limited range of motion.
- Maintain a straight upper body and avoid tilting to one side or the other.
- Throughout the workout, be mindful to keep your breathing under control.
- Try swinging your leg out to the side or circularly swinging both legs to make the workout more challenging.
- You may practice this exercise while standing close to a wall or counter for added stability if you have difficulties balancing.

Johnson Myers Ella

Extending Your Shoulders and Upper Body

Seniors may increase their flexibility and release stress in their upper bodies by stretching their shoulders and upper bodies. Here is a thorough example of how to carry out these stretches:

Start by taking a straight stance, placing your feet shoulder-width apart, and keeping your arms at your sides.

Reaching above your head with your right arm, place your hand on the left side of your head. Stretch your neck and shoulder by gently pulling your head to the right.

After 15 to 30 seconds of holding the stretch, release it and swap sides.

Next, extend your shoulder and upper back by placing your right hand on your left shoulder and gently pulling your elbow across your chest.

Johnson Myers Ella

After 15 to 30 seconds of holding the stretch, release it and swap sides.

To extend your chest and shoulders, clasp your hands behind your back and raise your arms over your head.

Release after 15–30 seconds of holding the stretch.

Advice and Changes:

- As your muscles warm up, start with moderate, easy stretches and progressively increase the intensity.
- Don't exert too much effort; stop if you experience pain or discomfort.
- Throughout the stretches, take calm, deep breaths to assist your muscles relax.
- Use a cloth or strap to aid extend your reach if you are unable to fully extend

your arms or shoulders during the stretch.

- Before doing these stretches, check with your doctor to be sure they are safe for you if you have any prior shoulder or upper body injuries or disorders.

Exercises With a Balance Board

Seniors may increase their flexibility and balance by engaging in entertaining and challenging balance board activities. A balancing board is a machine having a flat surface on top and a curved surface on the bottom, which may be used to do these exercises.

The unstable platform that the curved surface produces, tests the user's balance and works to build stronger balance-related muscles. An in-depth instruction on how a senior may do balance board exercises is below:

Johnson Myers Ella

Standing on the balancing board with your feet shoulder-width apart and your arms at your sides can help you develop fundamental balance.

Maintain a straight line of sight while concentrating on keeping your balance on the board. 30 seconds should be spent holding this posture before switching to the other foot.

On each foot, do this exercise 3–4 times. If necessary, use a chair or a wall as support. Work your way up to a smaller, more difficult board by beginning with a bigger, more sturdy board.

Standing on the balancing board with your feet shoulder-width apart and your arms at your sides, do lateral balance exercises. Lift the other foot off the board carefully and shift your weight to that foot. 30 seconds should be spent holding this posture before switching to the other foot. On each foot, do this exercise 3–4 times.

If necessary, use a chair or a wall as support. Work your way up to a smaller, more difficult board by beginning with a bigger, more sturdy board.

Single-Leg Balance

Put your hands by your sides while standing on the balancing board with your feet shoulder-width apart.

Put your weight on the foot you just carefully removed off the board. This position should be sustained for thirty seconds before switching to the other foot. On each foot, repeat this exercise three to four times.

If necessary, use a chair or a wall as support. Work your way down to a smaller, more difficult board after starting with a larger, more durable one.

Squats

Place your hands by your sides and stand on the balance board with your feet shoulder-width apart. Maintaining your balance on the board, slowly bend your knees and drop yourself into a squat. Holding this position for a few whiles, gently stand back up. Repeat this exercise a few more times.

If necessary, use a chair or a wall as support. Work your way down to a smaller, more difficult board after starting with a larger, more durable one.

Johnson Myers Ella

Modifications:

- Start with a larger, more stable board and work your way up to a smaller, more durable one.

- If necessary, use a chair or a wall as support.

- Reduce the time allotted for a workout or the number of repetitions if it is too difficult.

Stretching the Hamstrings

Any program for older citizens should include hamstring stretches to improve their balance and flexibility. Here is a comprehensive example of hamstring stretches for seniors, complete with advice and adjustments:

Stretch your legs out in front of you while sitting.

Your hands should be extended toward your toes as you progressively lean forward.

Stop when the back of your thighs starts to stretch. For 20 to 40 seconds, maintain this posture.
After releasing the stretch slowly, go back to the beginning position.

Stretching should be done two to three times, being cautious not to overexert oneself.

Tips:
- Refrain from exerting yourself. Stop after you feel a slight stretch, then start moving slowly and softly again.
- Throughout the stretch, maintain a straight back.
- Reach as far as you can without hurting yourself if you can't get to your toes.

Johnson Myers Ella

Modifications:

- Try sitting on a chair if you have problems sitting on the ground.

- Make use of a strap or piece of cloth to assist you if you are experiencing problems getting to your toes.

- If you have knee issues, stretch while keeping your knees slightly bent.

Flexing the Calf Muscles

Seniors may become more flexible and balanced while lowering their chance of injury by stretching their calves. Here is a thorough example of how a senior may perform calf stretches:

With your hands on the wall and your arms out in front of you, stand facing a wall.

Step forward with one foot, heel planted firmly and toes pointed forward.

Keep your back leg straight and firmly place your heel on the ground.

Once you feel the stretch in your calf muscle, hold the stretch for 20 to 40 seconds.
While relieving the strain, switch legs and move the other foot forward.

Maintain the stretch for 15 to 30 seconds on the opposing leg.

With breaks as necessary, the exercise should be performed in two to three sets.

Tips:

- Keep your back upright and avoid forward or waist bending.
- Don't force the stretch or bounce it. Hold it loosely at first and move slowly.

Johnson Myers Ella

- Stop stretching as soon as you experience any pain or discomfort.

Modifications:

- Move your front leg away from the wall and take a step backward to get a deeper stretch.

- Place a chair or other strong object nearby so you have something to grab onto if you have difficulties balancing.

- Before performing this exercise, see a physician or physical therapist if you are experiencing any knee or ankle issues.

Neck Exercises

Exercises for the neck may help seniors become more flexible and relieve tension in their upper back, shoulders, and neck. The following guidelines will show you how to properly do neck stretches as a workout to increase flexibility and balance:

Johnson Myers Ella

While you start, take a seat, put your hands on your thighs, and keep your feet flat on the ground.

As you gradually move your chin closer to your chest, you should feel a stretch at the back of your neck. Hold for 10 to 15 seconds, then slowly raise your head.

When your chin is almost touching your shoulder, try turning your head to the right. After then, slightly incline your head to the left. Hold for ten to fifteen seconds.

If you tilt your head to the right, your right ear will be near your right shoulder. Hold for 10 to 15 seconds, then slowly move your head to the left and repeat.

Johnson Myers Ella

Gently move your head around, starting with your chin in your chest, going to the right with your ear leaning toward your shoulder, and rolling until you are looking up at the ceiling. Continue once you take a new direction.

Advice and Alterations:

- Simply continue as far as you feel comfortable after starting slowly.
- Keep your neck's range of motion within reasonable bounds.
- If you have any neck injuries or pre-existing conditions, see a doctor or physical therapist before starting these exercises.
- Stop doing the stretches as soon as you experience any pain or discomfort and get medical help.

When conducting balance and flexibility exercises, it's crucial to begin softly and progressively increase their complexity over time. Seniors should contact their doctor before beginning any new fitness regimen, particularly if they have any health issues or concerns.

Chapter Three

Exercise Guidelines for Seniors

Here are some recommendations for older citizens to keep active and healthy via exercise:

Before beginning any fitness program, it is essential to speak with your healthcare physician, particularly if you have any current medical issues or concerns. Based on your unique health situation, your healthcare practitioner may provide tailored suggestions.

Pick a range of workouts, Cardiovascular activity, weight training, flexibility, and balancing exercises should all be a part of a well-rounded fitness program. Exercises that increase heart health and endurance include swimming, cycling, and walking. Maintaining muscle mass and bone density may be achieved by strength training using weights or resistance bands. Stretching and yoga are examples of flexibility activities that increase joint mobility and lower the risk of injury. Tai chi and other balance exercises assist to increase stability and lower the danger of falling.

If you've never exercised before or haven't been active in a while, it's crucial to start carefully and increase your activity level gradually. Start with low-intensity activities, and as your fitness level rises, progressively lengthen the frequency, and intensity of your workouts. Avoid pushing yourself too much and constantly pay attention to your body.

Practice appropriate form, using perfect form can help you avoid injuries and get the most out of your workouts. Consider working with a licensed physical therapist or fitness expert who

Johnson Myers Ella

can provide direction and training if you're uncertain about the proper technique.

Pay close attention to safety, seniors who exercise should put safety first. Exercise in a well-lit, well-ventilated place, and wear comfortable clothes and supportive footwear. If you need any assistive equipment, such as walking aids, use it. Stay hydrated, and stop exercising right away if you feel any pain, lightheadedness, or discomfort, and get help from a doctor if necessary.

Include rest and recovery, get enough rest and recuperation so that their bodies can heal and regenerate. Make sure to include rest days in your workout schedule, and if you start to feel tired or hurting, pay attention to your body.

Maintain consistency, exercise benefits must be attained and maintained over time. Strive to exercise often, preferably most days of the week. Even little bursts of movement throughout the day, like walking or completing tasks around the home, might be useful if you are unable to do lengthy workouts.

Maintain your social engagement, exercising is an excellent way to maintain your social engagement. To make exercise more fun and inspiring, think about signing up for group fitness programs, walking clubs, or participating in physical activities with friends or family.

Exercises should be modified as necessary since everyone has unique capabilities and limits. Exercises should be modified as necessary to accommodate your unique fitness level. Don't be hesitant to ask for advice from a fitness expert or healthcare practitioner.

Johnson Myers Ella

Lastly, constantly pay attention to your body, modify or stop the workout if anything doesn't feel correct or causes pain. It's crucial to exercise at a rate and level of difficulty that you find safe and satisfying.

Elders should exercise often to preserve their general health and well-being. You may maintain your health and fitness as you age by adhering to these workout recommendations. Prioritize safety, appropriate technique, and progressive development to ensure a safe and successful training regimen, and remember to always speak with your healthcare physician before beginning any exercise program.

Johnson Myers Ella

Johnson Myers Ella

Chapter Four

Conclusion

It is impossible to overestimate the advantages of exercise for elders over 60. The benefits of regular physical exercise on older individuals' physical, mental, and emotional health have been thoroughly documented. Exercise may help seniors maintain their muscular strength, flexibility, and balance, which are essential for avoiding falls and injuries, as we have discussed in this book. Additionally, it may promote mood and cognitive performance while lowering the risk of chronic illnesses including diabetes and osteoporosis.

It's crucial to keep in mind that it's never too late to start reaping the advantages of physical exercise for seniors who may be reluctant to do so. Even if you have spent a lot of time sitting

Johnson Myers Ella

still, adding a few easy workouts to your daily routine may have a positive impact on your health and quality of life. It's never too late to take control of your health and get the benefits of exercise.

To develop a customized fitness program that fits your unique requirements and medical issues, speak with your healthcare professional. There are also a ton of books, websites, and fitness plans created especially for seniors that provide advice on how to work out safely and effectively. Depending on your preferences and capabilities, you have a wide range of alternatives to select from, including walking and swimming as well as moderate yoga and chair exercises.

It's never too late to start adding regular exercise to your daily schedule. To develop a safe and efficient fitness program that meets your requirements, don't forget to talk to your healthcare practitioner and utilize the tools at your disposal. So, lace up your shoes, get a buddy for moral support, and start walking in the direction of a fitter, happier future!

www.ingramcontent.com/pod-product-compliance
Lightning Source LLC
Chambersburg PA
CBHW051827250726
48659CB00005B/1719